Paleo Diet for Weight Loss and Health

D1798649

Get Back to your Paleolithic Roots, Lose Massive Weight, and Become a Sexy Paleo Caveman or Cavewoman

Written by James Adler

Copyright © 2013,2016

www.HolisticWellnessBooks.com

My Paleo Experience

Are you tired of fad diets? Are you looking for a lifestyle transformation? Do you believe that **weight loss** is something more than getting slimmer? How about feeling **amazing** all the time, **radiating energy** and being a **health role model** to other people? If you are not a fan of extremely difficult and restrictive cleansings and fasts but would still like to **holistically detoxify your system**, you **have picked the right book**. It's not about some scientific mumbo jumbo- it's about **a practical approach** with **plenty of recipes to choose** from and fall in love with…it's not about torturing yourself for a few days and then giving up again and again (I have been there myself) but about shifting your focus and making a conscious decision **of body and mind transformation**.

Do you want to join me?

Ten years ago I was feeling ashamed when looking in the mirror. Now I feel proud. I know that it was hard work and dedication but it has totally paid off. I feel **energetic** and **literally bouncing off the walls**. I am 46 years old now and feel much fitter than when I was 20. Many people think that I am a professional athlete. I just tell them my story- **I transformed my body**. You can do it too. I really want to share my passion for **Paleo Diet** with other people and make it easy and doable for them.

My book explains the Paleo-perspective and ancient history behind the newest-oldest diet and how it is a multi-beneficial lifestyle change. The reason why this diet works is because it consists of **what we are biologically designed to eat**; what fuels our bodies to function properly for optimum health. It will show you not only how you can lose weight, gain energy you never thought you could have, and **cure/prevent a plethora of illnesses**.

Included are tips on how to start living Paleo, food lists, recipes, guidelines, and tools that will help you continue to live this way for the rest of your life.

I have always battled with my body in order to maintain a healthy weight. Some diets worked for a time, while others just failed from the beginning. I could lose 30 pounds but would gain it all back, if not more. In this book I am going to share my personal experience with you.

I was plagued with **allergies and asthma** from adolescence. The doctors always blamed my environment. During my late teens, I began experiencing **migraines**, depression, and anxiety. People told me that it was circumstantial, stress related, or just hormones.

About ten years ago, I noticed that an old friend of mine looked amazing. She was fit, looked bright and full of life, vibrant and healthy. She had suffered from many ailments all her life. I had to know, what was her secret? That is when I learned about Paleo diet. I dove right in and never looked back. It all coincided with other things that I attracted into my life: sport, yoga, meditation. I also started to study and investigated the field of nutrition and realized how brainwashed I became. We are constantly being sold an unhealthy lifestyle. Just analyze all the commercials, all over the world it is pretty much the same. We are all victims of the system where marketers very often try to sell what sells, not what is healthy and sustainable long-term. I felt amazed by my discovery.

Thanks to Paleo, I have maintained a weight loss of 40 pounds for nine years, have no allergy/asthma/migraine attacks, and my depression and anxiety are a thing of the past. It will work for you to... all you have to do is eat what we were biologically designed to consume.

This book is available as an audiobook, eBook and paperback.

You will find it in your local Amazon store, by looking for:

"James Adler Paleo Diet"

Enjoy!

DISCLAIMER

A physician has not written the information in this book. Although Paleo Diet is generally safe to use, you should consult your physician first to check if you can apply it. This book offers a general overview of the Paleo Diet to help you get started on it. For better results, I suggest you consult a dietician specialized in Paleo Diet. If you are suffering from severe obesity, I also suggest you consult with your physician.

Welcome Gift

Free Complimentary eBook

Before we dive into it, I would like to offer you a free complimentary eBook called: Alkaline Paleo Superfoods.

Simply visit:

www.holisticwellnessbooks.com/bonus to get your free copy now

As an added bonus, you will be notified about our new releases at discounted price, giveaways and a ton of useful health information to help you look and feel amazing.

Problems with your download?

Email us at: info@holisticwellnessbooks.com

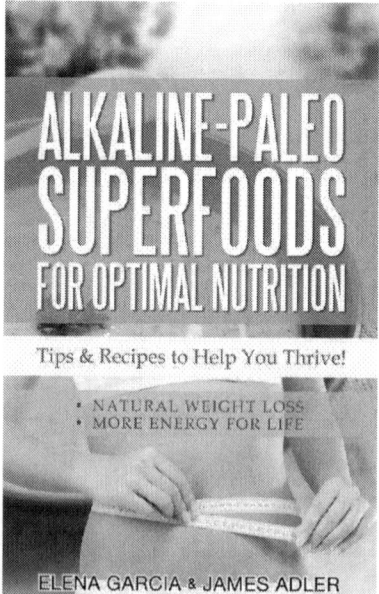

Table of Contents

Chapter 1 Paleo Lifestyle Made Easy

Are you looking for the newest, trendiest diet that uses fresh, new ideas and guiding principles to help you lose weight? Do you want to read up on the most contemporary, state of the art programs to get lean and energized? If you answered "yes," then the Paleo diet is NOT for you.

The Paleo diet is an approach to eating that originated a long time ago, during the Paleolithic era. This time frame started about 2.5 million years ago and ended around 10,000 years before our time. It avoids eating foods that only became part of the human diet after the agricultural revolution. The idea is that diseases like cancer and diabetes started around the same time that we began growing our own foods. The underlying principle is that the hunter-gatherers' diet is the reason they did not develop such diseases.

While we cannot be sure that their diet is what kept them healthy, there is enough research that concludes that foods banned from Paleo diets have little or no beneficial nutritional value. They have also been proven to interrupt normal hormonal balances, cause inflammation, and damage the lining of the gut. Eating Paleo will help to balance our bodies internally, protect the kidneys, protect the digestive tract from destructive proteins like gluten, and keep the liver and pancreas from having to work too hard.

Many names and titles have been given to this age-old eating program: the Paleolithic diet, Paleolithic nutrition, Paleo diet, Stone Age diet, caveman diet, and hunter-gatherer diet. Paleo Diet is an effort to go back to eating how we were biologically intended to eat. This method enables us to fuel our bodies properly so that they may function at their full genetic potential and start living healthier immediately. Foods that could be collected and consumed by hunting and gathering are what need to focus on. Primal eating at its best.

For me, I like to think of it as a Paleo perspective, not an actual diet. It could also be called a template. However you look at it, it is a lifestyle change. The goal is to eat like our ancestors did millions of years ago before the Agricultural Revolution.

Here are seven guidelines for Paleo nutrition that helped me to get a better idea of the principles involved in this primal nutritional practice.

1. Increase protein intake.

15% of the calories in most diets are from protein. When adhering to Paleo, that percentage must be much higher. It should be between 19-35 percent. A large amount of animal protein is required.

2. Decrease carbohydrate intake and eat foods lower on the glycemic index.

Most of the carbs will come from vegetables (and a few fruits). They should take up between 35-45 percent of your daily caloric intake. Most of the foods you will eat will be low on the glycemic index. They will not make your blood sugar spike because they are assimilated slowly.

3. Increase fiber consumption.

Paleos get their fiber from non-starchy vegetables. Vegetables such as these usually contain a fiber content around 30 percent higher than processed grain and about eight times higher than whole grain. Even fruits have more fiber than whole and refined grains.

4. **Increase fat intake by eating more monounsaturated and polyunsaturated fats.**

You need to do this in combination with a good balance of Omega-3 and Omega-6 fats. It is a common misconception that health is related to how *much* fat you eat, when the *type* of fat you eat affects your health more. Increase monounsaturated and Omega-3 fats and remove Trans and Omega-6 polyunsaturated fats.

5. **Raise potassium while lowering sodium.**

Paleolithic humans consumed foods that were unrefined and fresh. Potassium levels in fresh foods are between 5-10 percent higher than sodium levels. Potassium helps the heart, kidneys, and other organs function correctly. People who have low potassium levels are more susceptible to elevated blood pressure, stroke, and cardiovascular disease. Excessive sodium levels can also cause the same problems. Many modern diets contain two times as much sodium as potassium.

6. **Eat more alkaline than acidic foods.**

When we consume food, it has either an acid or alkaline effect on your body. Even on a Paleo diet, it is necessary to keep this in mind because meat and fish are both acid-forming foods. Alkaline-producing foods include most vegetables and fruits. Having an acidic system for a long time can lead to atrophy of the muscles and bone, elevated blood pressure, kidney stones, and can trigger things like asthma and allergies.

7. Increase the intake of vitamins, phytochemicals, minerals, and antioxidants.

Whole grains are a poor source of these things. The few minerals and vitamins that are actually in whole grains are not usually processed and absorbed properly by the body. They do not contain vitamin C, A, or B12. There truly is no substitute for grass-produced and free-range meat or organic vegetables and fruits.

What foods did the cavemen eat? What foods did they hunt, and what did they go out and gather? These are two key questions to keep in mind when deciding what to eat on the Paleo diet.

Basic categories of foods to consume when eating Paleo:

➢ Grass-produced meats

➢ Fish and seafood

➢ Eggs

➢ Fresh fruits and vegetables

➢ Seeds

➢ Healthful oils (olive, walnut, flaxseed, macadamia, avocado, or coconut)

The foods included on the Paleo diet are foods that our cave-dwelling ancestors would have access to on a regular basis.

Basic categories of what NOT to eat when eating Paleo:

➢ Cereals and grains

➢ Potatoes

- Legumes

- Sugars

- Processed foods

- Salt

- Dairy

- Refined vegetable oil

Some people do not understand exactly what a legume is. A legume is the seed pod of a plant that is edible. Examples of legumes are:

- Beans

- Peas

- Lentils

- Peanuts

- Alfalfa

- Clover

- Carob

- Soy

- Lupini

Essentially, if a caveman could not have eaten it 10,000 years ago, you cannot eat it now. No consuming packaged foods at all. If it contains chemicals or ingredients that you cannot pronounce, then it is probably not Paleo.

Chapter 2 Losing Weight with Paleo

Eating a Paleo diet takes us back to basics. Way back. You may be wondering, "If this 'diet' is so old, why am I only just hearing about it?" Buzz is being generated because people are stepping away from modern eating habits and feeling better. Paleo nutritional practices are helping people lose weight, have tons of energy, lessen inflammation, clear up skin problems, gain muscle, cure allergies, stop asthma symptoms, get rid of digestive issues, get people off of their diabetes medicines, and much more.

As I stated previously, I did not just want to lose weight by eating Paleo. I had a variety of other health problems: headaches, asthma, allergies, anxiety, depression, and acne. Paleolithic nutrition can aid you in ridding yourself of these illnesses along with countless others. Eating Paleo also means preventing Alzheimer's, diabetes, cardiovascular disease, and cancer. All of these problems have a common contributing factor: inflammation.

LOSING WEIGHT - MY PERSONAL EXPERIENCE

How did adopting the Paleo lifestyle help me lose weight? Easy answer: carbs, calories, caffeine, and my immune system. In order to see how it worked, I needed to know why I ended up getting/being fat in the first place.

1) Eating too many calories causes weight gain.

When eating refined, processed carbs (bread, crackers, chips, rice, cookies, etc.), it is very easy to eat too many calories, which leads to weight gain. These foods are full of calories, but will not fill you up. That is how we sometimes end up eating too much. These refined carb and calorie-dense foods will spike blood sugar, but what goes up will come down, and we are left with a crash in blood sugar. Most of the time, it makes you think that you want to eat sweets minutes later because the brain wants the blood sugar to spike again. I know that all too often, I have eaten a bowl of spaghetti and garlic bread only to be starving a half hour later!

Protein and fat have been proven to be more filling foods than refined carbohydrates. Meats and fats help to ensure that I do not over eat. They keep me fuller for a longer period of time than rice or bread. If you eat 300 calories worth of chicken, you will feel fuller longer than if you ate 300 calories worth of chips.

I no longer snack on calorie-rich foods that leave me hungry for more. I eat three or four meals full of protein and fats in combination with fibrous, nutrient-rich vegetables and fruit. I feel full for hours and consume significantly fewer calories. I no longer have to drink coffee all day long because my blood sugar levels are a lot more stable and my foods are nutrient-rich. I get enough energy from my diet alone!

2) Drinking caffeine can make you fat.
Caffeine is a stimulant that creates a highly stressful state in your body. This stress from caffeine encourages your body to create cortisol. Cortisol can upset digestive processes and causes fat to accumulate around the middle body.

Although I did not notice at the time, I was drinking caffeine because processed grains were making me lethargic. They can have an effect on the body that is the equivalent of taking an opiate. Blood sugar crashes are also to blame. Sure, there was the occasional late night when I needed a pick-me-up the next morning, but the major cause of my caffeine consumption was due to the grains in my diet.

After removing foods that sent my blood sugar on a roller-coaster ride every day, I stopped needing caffeine. Those grain-induced comatose moments were also gone, so the need to counter-act them with copious amounts of caffeine was no longer there, either.

3) My immune system was making me fat.

Wheat, soy, grains, and beans contain anti-nutrients that are impossible for our bodies to digest. They contain these elements to deter plants' natural predators from eating them. The result of eating and trying to digest them is digestive distress in the form of gas, bloating, diarrhea, and worse. All of these results are things people have come to accept as part of eating. Yet, these symptoms are indications that what we are eating is unnatural in relation to digestion.

What could be worse, you might ask? Well, those anti-nutrients can stick to the lining of the intestine and cause it to break down. Food particles escape the intestine and get into the blood stream in a condition called "leaky gut." This causes your immune system to respond to the invader and try to fight it. This can cause eczema, headaches, water retention, inflammation, and other nasty things.

I cannot stand water retention. It adds to the feeling of being fat. It adds weight, makes you appear larger in general, and makes your stomach feel bloated.

After I removed the grains and legumes that contain anti-nutrients from my diet, my intestines were able to slowly heal. My immune system calmed down. My water retention went away. Eating Paleo was the key.

Taking on a Paleo nutritional perspective allowed me to lose weight, and better yet, keep it off. I no longer ate calorie-rich foods that left me wanting more. I no longer needed to drink caffeine to get through my day. My immune system stopped going crazy because my intestines had time to heal. Sure, I lost a lot of variety in convenience foods, but I gained a more energetic, healthy, slim self.

CURING MY OTHER AILMENTS

Inflammation is the body's natural response to invaders. I already discussed this problem and how "leaky gut" will lead to weight gain. It may be more important to note that "leaky gut" will lead to major health issues because it causes chronic inflammation. Cancer, asthma, headaches, allergies, arthritis, auto-immune disorders, heart disease, diabetes, depression, Alzheimer's, and osteoporosis are all caused by chronic inflammation. The list goes on and on.

Why does inflammation cause so many problems? Inflammation is an immune system response. It is used by the body to battle intruders that are unidentified or already deemed harmful. Well, how could something good cause such a problem? Let me explain it this way. It is like leaving the heater turned up and the thermostat not working. It never turns off when the environment gets to a certain temperature. Yes, you wanted to warm up, but if it never turns off, it will get way too hot. It will negatively affect whatever is in the environment.

Converting to a Paleolithic nutritional lifestyle has allowed me to eat a diet that is void of inflammatory foods. Aside from healing "leaky gut," thus allowing the immune system to calm down, Paleo diets also reduce inflammation in many other ways. I have highlighted a few below:

> The diet is high in vitamin D. Vitamin D has been proven to aid in reducing inflammation.

> The diet is high in phytonutrients, many of which have anti-inflammatory effects.

> The immune system reacts to factors in the environment that it has been exposed to (pollen, bacteria, molds, etc.) with inflammation. The Paleo diet has the effect of making the immune system less prone to react to these factors and also makes it more effective because it is not over-loaded.

> The Paleo perspective adjusts the Omega-3/Omega-6 proportion to a beneficial ratio and makes it an effective agent in battling inflammatory illnesses. An Omega-3/6 imbalance can result from eating vegetable oils, grain products, and a deficiency of DHA and EPA from animal products.

Yes, I wanted to lose weight and reduce fat by adopting my new lifestyle. I was also looking to get rid of the ailments and issues that had been with me most of my adolescent and adult life. Paleolithic nutrition made this happen for me, and it can help you in countless areas of your life and health as well.

Chapter 3 How to Get Started?

I am frequently asked what steps I took when I first started eating under the Paleo guidelines. Just *starting* the Paleo program is essentially the most difficult part. Learning about the benefits of Paleo, what and what not to eat, and how it works is a great pre-game strategy, but it is not an actual step into this prolific nutritional lifestyle.

Purging all of the non-Paleo foods from our lives seems to be the hardest part, so I recommend diving right in and doing that first. These foods have been so ingrained into our lifestyles and culture (not to mention that some are physically addictive) that it is hard to think about living without them. That is why we have to focus on the underlying principle of the Paleo diet: in order to achieve optimum health, we need to eat as our ancient ancestors did. They lived without any of these foods, and so can we.

The unhealthy food that is in your kitchen will be eaten if you leave it there. These foods are quick to prepare and easier to make than healthy Paleo meals. When I am hungry, it is much faster to open a box of crackers or make some Ramen noodles than it is to prepare a healthy, fresh Paleo meal. Keep your kitchen free of unhealthy foods and packed full of nutrient-rich fresh foods. I did this first. By removing all of the temptations, it was easier to make the good stuff and more difficult to consume the bad stuff.

WHAT TO REMOVE

These are not complete lists, of course, but they will give you a general idea of what to get rid of and what not to forget. Basically, throw out everything in a box, wrapper, or bag. Usually, if it has more than 3 ingredients or if you cannot pronounce the ingredients, it needs to be removed from the premises. When you're unsure about a certain item, better safe than sorry. Just toss it!

Pantry: Chips, pretzels, tortillas, baked goods, peanuts, instant foods, cereal, bread, bagels, pasta, any mixes, canned beans, crackers, granola bars, rice, sugar, anything processed, etc.

Freezer: Ice cream, frozen breakfast foods, pizzas, hot dogs, candy, etc.

Fridge: Processed meats, dairy, juice, all alcoholic beverages, anything sweetened, leftovers, margarine, breads, whole wheat products, condiments, peanut butter, etc.

WHAT TO BUY NOW:

After I got rid of everything in my kitchen that would deter my goal of eating cave-man/woman style, I had to replenish my fridge and cupboards with produce and meats that would complement my new lifestyle.

Sticking to the aisles around the perimeter of the store is usually a good idea when shopping at any kind of grocery store. I had never realized it before, but that is where all the fresh produce, fruit, and animal protein is located. There are also many detailed Paleo food lists that you can print out online. I still keep one in my purse to this day, just in case.

Reading labels is a must-do for any Paleo dieter. For the most part, anything with a label is probably something you do not want to buy. If it does have a label, but you can't pronounce the ingredients, do not purchase it. Here are some things that I keep in mind when I grocery shop:

Best = Zero ingredients

Better = One ingredient

Ok = Two ingredients

Pushing my luck = Three ingredients

No way = Four+ ingredients

Key words to remember when shopping to stock a Paleo kitchen: Organic, grass-fed, pasture-raised, wild-caught, free-range, and raw.

I had to replace everything in my pantry with new ingredients that I would be using in Paleo recipes. I had previewed these new recipes, and if you are anything like me, these ingredients sounded strange. They are staples of the Paleo kitchen and will benefit you in preparing many delicious Paleo meals and snacks. This a list of items that are usually used in Paleo recipes:

- **Blanched almond flour**

- **Coconut flour**

- **Almond meal**

- **Extra virgin coconut Oil**

- **Refined coconut oil**

- **Palm shortening**

- **Arrowroot powder/Tapioca starch**

- **Ground flax meal**

- **Coconut milk**

- **Creamed coconut**

- **Unsweetened coconut flakes**

- **Unsweetened shredded coconut**

- **Nuts**: Whole almonds, pecan halves, walnut halves, macadamia nuts, hazelnuts, pistachios, cashews, Brazil nuts

- **Almond Butter**

- **Raw/natural cocoa powder**

- **Honey**

- **Raw maple syrup**

- **Leavening/Spices**: Baking soda, cream of tartar, allspice, cinnamon, salt, cloves, cardamom, ground ginger, nutmeg, vanilla extract, vanilla bean, lemon juice

As for my refrigerator, I stock it with plenty of grass-feed, free-range, organic meats, wild-caught fish, and tons of Paleo-approved fresh produce.

The next thing I had to consider when I began this lifestyle was that I needed to **start cooking** all of **my own food**. No more convenience foods or fast food. I started gathering recipes for quick meals that could be prepared during the week. I started making large meals that would leave lots of leftovers. These leftovers will be your new convenience foods. You can fill your freezer with home-cooked meals that can be reheated quickly on busy days.

Now, aside from the kitchen, there are two other areas of my lifestyle that needed to be addressed when I was starting this primal lifestyle: sleep and the dreaded detox.

SLEEP

Getting enough sleep was probably not very difficult for our hunter-gatherer ancestors. For us, it is much more difficult thanks to a toxic diet and the invention of electricity. These two things have left us in a state of sleep deprivation.

Sleep deprivation can cause many problems including weight gain, hormonal imbalances, heart disease, lowered immune system function, long periods of high cortisone levels, and many more.

If you do not sleep enough, you may have difficulty in resisting sugary foods that will sabotage your new healthy lifestyle. Eating these carb-filled sugary foods will ruin your sleep schedule because they change your blood sugar levels. Sleep is a key component of successfully adopting the Paleo lifestyle.

Sleep works together with a nutritious Paleo diet to help the body function at its best. Here are some tips that I used in order to get enough sleep.

1. **I went to bed at the same time every night.**

2. **I made sure that my bedroom was super dark with no lights at all.**

3. **I made sure that my bedroom had proper air circulation.**

4. **I cut out all caffeine.**

5. **I did not drink alcohol.**

6. **I made sure that I was in bed by 10 p.m. and out of bed by 7 a.m.**

7. **I was up when the sun was up.**

8. **I stayed away from using any electronics 2 hours before bed and made sure that no electronics were plugged in near my bed.**

Getting enough sleep helped me to stay strong when facing temptation at the start of my new ancient eating program. It also helped me feel more energized throughout the day while my body adjusted to using fat as an energy source.

I found natural therapies to be very helpful in my case. They helped me restore healthy sleep patterns and rejuvenate myself. Getting enough healthy sleep will prevent you from overeating or indulging in unhealthy foods.

THE DREADED DETOX

For about 2-3 weeks (maybe longer) when people first start the Paleo diet, most feel tired, frail, and unproductive. I had the same experience. My body was dependent upon sugars and starches for energy. When I removed them, my body went into shock. It takes a while for your body to learn how to use fat as an energy source. The body is also releasing toxins during this time; toxins that have been building up for a very long time. Fight the urges to give into caffeine and sugar. Stay away from grains. This feeling will not last forever.

After this time period passed, I began to notice that something wonderful was happening inside my body. I felt energized for most of the day. I was not constantly hungry. I was not craving the sugars and refined carbs, nor was I craving the whole grain foods. I felt amazing and wondered why I had never done this before. I craved real, whole, energizing, fresh foods. I had done it, and there was no turning back.

The first move to make when implementing the Paleo way of life is simply getting started. When? I say right now. Today is one more day you could have spent getting your body healthy. It only takes minutes to perform a kitchen overhaul. I went straight to the store afterward and was preparing my first Paleo meal in hours. Why would you delay when the future looks bright?

Chapter 4 Basic Paleo Recipes for Weight Loss and Vitality

I love to cook. Paleo cooking is fun because you can mix and match so many different things to create many different meals. Experimenting with different meat, herb, oil, and vegetable combinations is exciting. Of course, everyone loves a good recipe, and I will provide some of my favorites.

People who practice Paleo living usually benefit from meal planning. This enables you to have the items you will need for the week on hand. Cooking Paleo meals usually requires mostly fresh ingredients. By planning ahead, you will know everything you will need to get in one trip to the store.

Here are a few tips for Paleo meal planning:

1. Make certain to eat a lot of vegetables. Eating Paleo does not mean eat more meat than anything else. Eating vegetables is key.

2. Make sure the meat you are eating are lean cuts, not processed meat.

3. Pay attention to how much fat you are consuming and confirm that you are eating enough of it every day. A clue that you are not getting enough fat is that you are always hungry or never feel all the way full. If this is the case, eat more avocado or coconut.

4. Try new things. Experimenting with Paleo is fun. Use a meat or vegetable that you have never heard of before. Try a combination that seems unlikely. You may love it!

5. Do not shy away from bacon. Eat plenty of it, it goes with almost everything.

Every day you will be eating breakfast, lunch, dinner, and a snack. I appreciate that in Paleo, breakfasts can be anything, they don't have to be "breakfast." Leftovers make a quick breakfast solution. Here a couple of my favorite morning breakfasts, mid-day lunches, and evening dinners. Enjoy!

BREAKFAST

#1. Pan-caves

Servings - 1

Ingredients:

- 1 cup almond flour

- 1 egg

- ⅔ cup almond milk

- Washed strawberries

- Washed blueberries

- 1 banana

- ½ cup almond flakes

Instructions:

1. Heat a pan to medium heat. When warm, add almond flakes to toast them. When they are toasted, add strawberries and blueberries and heat. Allow the berries to soften up.

2. Put the mixture into a bowl and set aside.

3. Whisk the egg, flour, and milk in a bowl until smooth. If it appears runny, add a spoonful of almond flour.

4. Reheat the pan to high heat with a bit of oil.

5. Pour batter into the pan, moving it around a bit.

6. It should start to brown around the edges and firm up, then flip.

7. Repeat steps 4-6 until you have used all your batter.

8. Top with the toasted almond/berry mixture.

Serve with bacon! Enjoy!

#2. Easy Paleo Scramble

<u>Servings - 2 to 3</u>

<u>Ingredients:</u>

- 6 eggs

- 1 poblano pepper

- 1 onion

- ⅔ cup mushrooms

- ½ cup tomatoes

- 2 cups cooked ham

<u>Instructions:</u>

1. Chop pepper, onion, mushrooms, tomato, and ham.

2. Cook the pepper and onion in coconut oil or bacon grease over medium heat until onion is clear.

3. Next, add the mushrooms, tomatoes, and ham in the same pan and cook until the ham has browned.

4. Lastly, crack the eggs into the pan, scramble with the veggies and tomato until eggs are done. Season to taste.

#3. Spinach and Brussels Frittata

Servings - 3 to 4

Ingredients:

- 8 eggs, whisked
- 2 cups Brussels sprouts, cut in fourths
- 5-6 cups fresh spinach
- 3 tablespoons bacon fat
- 2 garlic cloves, minced
- 1 tsp. garlic powder
- ½ teaspoon paprika
- Salt and pepper
- Avocado to garnish

Instructions:

Preheat oven to 375 degrees.

1. Heat bacon fat or a few tablespoons of coconut oil in a skillet over medium-high heat. Once heated, add garlic, Brussels sprouts, salt, and pepper. Cook until they brown on one side, then flip sprouts to ensure that they brown on all sides (takes approximately five minutes).

2. Add the spinach and put a lid on so that it will steam. Cook for 4 more minutes until the spinach is soft.

3. In a separate bowl, whisk eggs, garlic powder, and seasonings. When the vegetables are done, mix them into the egg mixture.

4. Pour the egg/vegetable mixture into a large baking dish or cast iron skillet.

5. Put in preheated oven for 15-18 minutes, depending how big the skillet is. Check to make sure it is done by pressing on the middle. If it is done, it will push back. Top with avocado. Enjoy!

LUNCH

#4. Spicy Tuna with Artichokes

<u>Servings - 2</u>

<u>Ingredients:</u>

- 2 tbsp. coconut oil

- 1/2 red onion (sliced as thinly as possible)

- Artichoke hearts (however many you like)

- 1 lemon, sliced

- 2 cloves of garlic, sliced

- 4 sprigs fresh thyme

- 1 ½ lb. fresh tuna (1 inch cubes)

- 1 ½ tsp. sea salt

- 1 tsp. black pepper

- 1 tsp. cayenne pepper

- 3-4 cups steamed veggies

<u>Instructions:</u>

1. Heat 1 tbsp. of oil and sauté onions for about 3 minutes. Throw in artichoke hearts, lemon, garlic, and thyme. Cook for about three more minutes, then set aside.

2. Season tuna. Heat the rest of the oil in the same skillet and brown the tuna on all sides. Cook to your liking.

3. Add the artichokes, lemon, garlic and thyme to the tuna and mix together. Serve and enjoy!

#5.Guacamole Peppers

Servings - 2 to 3

Ingredients:

- 5 small/medium poblano peppers

- 2 ripe avocados, cut in half and pits removed

- ¼ cup chopped fresh cilantro

- ¼ cup finely chopped red onion

- ¼ teaspoon salt

- 1 cup shredded hearts of romaine

Instructions:

Preheat broiler on High.

1. Put peppers on a broiler pan or cookie sheet. Broil 3 to 4 inches below the heat. Turn a couple of times until the skins blacken and bubble (10 minutes or so). Put in a bowl, cover, and let stand 10-15 minutes. They will be easy to peel now. Leave stems attached.

2. Scoop avocados into a bowl and mash with a fork. Stir in cilantro, onion, and salt.

3. Stem and seed one of the peppers and chop. Mix it into the guacamole.

4. Make a slit through one wall of each of the remaining 4 peppers top to bottom and remove seeds. Put romaine in each of the peppers, then fill with a generous 1/3 cup guacamole each.

#6. Mexican Chicken Salad

<u>Servings - 4</u>

<u>Ingredients:</u>

CHICKEN:
- 1 lb. boneless, skinless chicken breasts
- 1 tbsp. oil of your choice
- Salt and pepper

SALSA:
- 1 large tomato, quartered
- ½ red onion, cut into large pieces
- 1 jalapeño pepper, stem and seeds removed and halved
- 1 clove of garlic
- 1 small bunch of cilantro leaves
- 1 lime (to squeeze juice from)
- Salt and pepper

<u>Instructions:</u>

Preheat oven to 375.

1. Lightly coat chicken breasts in olive oil and season. Bake in oven 35 to 40 minutes.

2. Chop all salsa ingredients in a food processor or by hand.

3. Take chicken out of the oven. Once it cools, cut up the chicken and throw into the food processor. Pulse until shredded (or you can shred it with a fork).

4. Mix together chicken and salsa.

5. Refrigerate salad until it is chilled.

Serve over greens of your choice. Enjoy!

DINNER

#7. Zucchini Chicken

Servings - 3 to 4

Ingredients:

- 2 tbsp. coconut oil

- 8 chicken drumsticks

- Sea salt and pepper

- 1 tbsp. poultry seasoning

- 1 yellow onion, cut into large pieces

- 4 cloves garlic (chopped or minced)

- 1 cup tomatoes (diced)

- 5 small zucchinis, cut into large pieces

Instructions:

Heat coconut oil in a sauce pan. Season drumsticks and add to pan. Brown on all sides.

Sprinkle poultry seasoning over the drumsticks. Add the diced tomatoes, onion, and garlic.

Simmer over medium-low heat for 15-20 minutes.

Now, add the zucchini. Continue to cook over medium-low heat for an additional 5 minutes.

Enjoy! I do!

#8. Bacon-topped Meatloaf

<u>Servings - 3</u>

<u>Ingredients:</u>

- 2 lb. Grass Fed ground beef

- 1 lb. ground pork

- 2 organic eggs

- 1 cup almond flour

- 1 cup tomato sauce

- 12 slices of bacon (nitrate free)

- 1 onion, chopped

- 2 15 oz. tomatoes, roasted under broiler, skins and seeds removed

- 1 cup roasted red peppers

- 5 cloves of garlic

- 1 tsp. cumin

- 1 tsp. oregano

<u>Instructions:</u>

1. Preheat oven to 350 degrees

2. Mix 1 of the tomatoes, roasted red peppers, garlic, cumin, and oregano in a food processor. Mix the pork, onions, beef, almond flour, eggs, and tomatoes in a large bowl.

3. Place into a baking pan (large loaf pan), then salt and pepper.

4. Top with bacon and cook for 45 minutes.

5. Turn broiler on and cook for an additional 10 minutes.

6. Simmer the rest of the tomatoes in a sauce pan for 15 minutes.

7. When the meatloaf is done, top with the simmered tomato sauce.

8. Serve with sautéed kale (see below)

Enjoy!

#9 Sautéed Kale

<u>Servings - 2</u>

<u>Ingredients:</u>

- 2 tbsp. olive or coconut oil

- 1 large onion chopped

- 1 bunch kale cut into 1-inch strips

- ¼ teaspoon sea salt

<u>Instructions:</u>

1. Heat oil over medium heat.

2. Reduce heat to medium-low and add onion.

3. Sauté for 15 minutes or until onions have caramelized.

4. Put kale in the pan with the onions and sauté for 5 minutes uncovered.

5. Cover pot with a lid and cook for 1-2 minutes so that kale is completely wilted.

6. Add salt

Enjoy!

#10. One Dish Fish

<u>Servings - 4</u>

<u>Ingredients:</u>

- 4 fish fillets (about 1 ½ lbs.) Salmon, tilapia, cod (or a mix)

- 1 cup of cherry tomatoes

- 2 yellow squash

- 2 green bell pepper

- ¼ cup olive oil

- 1 tbsp. apple cider vinegar

- 1 tbsp. vodka or gin

- Salt and pepper

- 1 tbsp. tamari soy sauce, coconut aminos, or Bragg's liquid aminos

<u>Instructions:</u>

Preheat oven to 375F.

1. Chop up the fish, squash, and bell pepper into 1-inch cubes.
2. Put all ingredients into a large casserole dish.
3. Bake for 35 minutes uncovered.

Enjoy!

I included very simple, delicious Paleo recipes in order to prove that Paleo cooking does not need to be complicated. I started out with these same recipes. There are many out there to choose from. I sometimes enjoy turning my favorite Neolithic recipes into recipes that fit my Paleo nutritional perspective. I also love coming up with original recipes. It is my hope that the recipes I shared with you will show you that Paleo cooking is fun and easy! Carry on reading to discover more.

Chapter 5 Paleo Healthy Snacks: How to Avoid Cheating

In a perfect world, snacking in the Paleo lifestyle would be unnecessary. You would always be able to eat the perfect sized meal, packed with the appropriate nutrients that would keep you feeling full until the next one. Well, the world is not perfect, and even those who achieve Paleo-perfection sometimes need something to tide them over. Situations like this call for us to have pre-planned snack options to keep us on track.

These snacks are especially important for Paleo-newbies in their first 3-4 weeks to keep them on the right track during moments of weakness. Here are 10 snacks that are easily prepared and some crisis snacks to keep on hand just in case.

1) Roasted Pumpkin Seeds

Full of potassium, fiber, and protein, pumpkin seeds are easy to make and delicious. Just heat the oven to 350, coat the seeds in coconut oil, and spread them on a baking sheet. Put them in for around 20 minutes until they are golden brown, and be sure to stir them halfway. I add cayenne pepper, but you can add almost any spice or seasoning.

2) Tuna and Avocado

They are both super good for you and include protein and healthy fat to keep you full! Just scoop out the avocado into a bowl and mix in some tuna and a big squeeze of lemon! I add cayenne and pepper, but season as you would like.

3) Kale Chips

My absolute favorite! They are super healthy and can help when you want something to munch.

Here is the mini recipe:

- Preheat oven to 350 degrees Fahrenheit (175 Celsius)
- Tear up kale put into a bowl. Drizzle with avocado or coconut oil.
- Bake for twelve minutes. Remove and sprinkle with your favorite seasoning. SO delicious.

4) Good ol' Bacon and Eggs

Use a muffin tray and put 2 bacon strips in each cup, then crack an egg inside. Preheat oven to 350 and bake for 10 minutes.

5) Veggies and Paleo Hummus

Raw veggies can kill the urge to munch, and hummus is never a bad idea!

Zucchini Hummus
- 2 medium zucchinis, peeled and cut into large pieces
- ½ cup tahini
- ⅓ cup lemon juice
- ⅓ cup extra virgin olive oil
- 3 cloves garlic
- 2 teaspoons cumin
- Salt & pepper (add cayenne if you like it spicy)

Put everything except oil into the food processer. Slowly add oil until well-combined and smooth.

EMERGENCY SNACKS

6) Fresh fruit

Always have it washed and ready to eat!

7) Cut vegetables

Curbs snack cravings and are good to have on hand for meals and salads as well. I cut a full bags worth of each on grocery day! Truly a lifesaver.

8) Fresh cold sliced meats

A typical Paleo snack idea, but you would be surprised how many people do not think of it. Make sure the brand is Paleo-friendly.

9) Trail mix of nuts and seeds

Mix up your favorites and keep in a container in the pantry. When I know I may be out and about, I throw a handful in a snack-sized baggie.

10) A can of tuna

Keep them on hand in the cupboard or the fridge. Always a winner.

These snacks will help to keep you from cheating. The options are almost endless, but it is always good to have a list to start with, and these are my favorites. They will also help you not feel so hungry and fall off of the Paleo wagon easily. The more you see Paleo working for you, the more you will work for it!

Chapter 6 Awesome Paleo Recipes - Back to the Cave!

What was the biggest obstacle in my Paleo dieting adventure? Lack of variety. I got stuck eating the same stuff over and over again, and I would automatically go back to my old unhealthy eating patterns simply because I felt like I was missing something. Then I realized that it takes some time to become Paleo-creative. First, you need guidance — more and more Paleo friendly recipes to keep on track.

This is why I am adding this next chapter, which will provide you with plenty of super-healthy and delicious Paleo recipes for the whole family to enjoy.

Make it easy for yourself and don't make the same mistakes that I was making. There is no point in going back to where you were before.

It's up to you if you decide to do your Paleo thing full-time or part-time. For example, my wife, Elena, is a big fan of the alkaline diet. In fact, we have a free PDF e-book you can get at:

www.holisticwellnessbooks.com/bonus

My suggestion is to prepare your weekly menus on Sundays. Plan your shopping list, food for work, snacks, Paleo treats, and dinners that you can have with friends. Invite them over and get them addicted to this amazing diet!

The previous chapter was merely an introduction for beginners. You will find many more Paleo recipes here.

Ok, ladies and gentlemen, it's time to get back to the CAVE with the following recipes.

#12 Yummy Paleo Cake

Servings - 5

Ingredients:

- 250g (1 cup) raw almonds
- 70g (¼ cup) agave syrup
- Zest of a lemon (you can use 2 lemons as well)
- 4 organic eggs (make sure they are organic and free-range)
- Olive oil (coconut oil works too, if you are a coconut oil lover!)
- Eco-dark chocolate 100% cacao

Preparation:

1. Preheat oven to 180°C (355°F).

2. Crush almonds and set aside in a small bowl.

3. Whisk the lemon peel, agave, and eggs.

4. Add crushed almonds and stir.

5. Grease an oven-safe pan with olive or coconut oil (around 1 tbsp.).

6. Pour the paleo batter into the pan, then put in the oven. Bake for about 15-20 minutes.

7. Remove from the oven and serve with organic chocolate on top.

8. Enjoy! I always do!

#13 Veggies in a Cave

My wife absolutely loves this dish. I think she was born to be a vegetarian. Now, many people think that the Paleo Diet is only about eating meat in exaggerated amounts. I think that it's all about finding balance. So, have no fear when you see a nice plate of fresh vegetables. Of course, if your salivary glands are looking for something meaty, or you are an athlete, you can add some bacon or tuna as well. However, aside from my Paleo preferences, I am also a firm believer in the Alkaline Diet. Hence, I like to detoxify my body and go alkaline from time to time.

Servings - 2 to 3

Prep time - 15 minutes

Ingredients

- 1 onion
- 2 zucchinis
- 8 mushrooms
- 4 asparagus
- 1 leek
- Condiments: coarse salt, cumin, and olive oil.

PREPARATION:

1. Wash and chop the vegetables into small or medium-sized pieces.

2. Put on the grill (I use one that does not require using any kind of oil for cooking) set to low heat.

3. Add salt and cumin. Flip occasionally so that your veggies don't burn themselves to death (it takes about 10-15 minutes on low heat).

4. Remove when ready and add a drizzle of olive oil to the plate.

OPTIONAL: Add some bacon or tuna to your veggie mix. You can also use algae (more on algae later)

This recipe is a mix of paleo diet and alkaline diet.

Remember to get your free PDF eBook that will help you get the best of paleo and alkaline lifestyle, to create a holistic diet that works for you:

www.HolisticWellnessBooks.com/bonus

#14. Alkaline Paleo Soup

Here comes another light veggie dish. Again, paleo is not only about eating meat.

Servings - 4

Ingredients:

- 1 stalk of broccoli (500 grams, or around 2 cups)
- 4 medium onions
- 4 cloves of garlic
- Curry, sea salt, and olive oil

Prep Time: 20 minutes

PREPARATION:

1. Put the chopped broccoli, chopped onions, garlic, and a few tablespoons of salt in a pan with a pint of water. Heat to medium.

2. When everything is slightly boiling, add some curry. Cook for about 2 minutes while stirring and turn off.

3. Drain the water into a bowl. Set aside a few pieces of broccoli for later to garnish the dish when it's ready.

4. Add a splash of olive oil and blend the veggies. Add some more salt and oil if needed (taste it first)

5. Serve in bowls, place a piece of broccoli in the center, and add a drizzle of olive oil on top.

I also like using coconut oil with this recipe. It gives the soup really nice, creamy taste!

Irresistible. It's cool to be healthy, right?

Of course, you can also add some bacon or chicken.

#15 Salmon Rocks!

I can never get fed up with salmon. It is a great source of healthy fats and gives me all the protein I need to for paleo athletic endeavors! My wife also likes it, she is not a big fan of meat, but she absolutely loves fish.

Servings - 2

Prep Time: 15 minutes

Ingredients

- 6 free-range organic eggs

- 6 mushrooms

- 6 medium artichoke hearts

- 100g smoked salmon

- 4 cloves garlic

- Salt and olive oil (Optional: I also like some rosemary in this recipe.)

PREPARATION:

1. Chop the garlic into small pieces and start frying slightly in a little oil. Keep the heat low.

2. Add the mushrooms (finely chopped) and artichokes. You may also want to add a pinch of salt.

3. When the juices start coming out of the veggies, add salmon (chopped in small pieces)

4. Add the beaten eggs, stirring with a wooden spatula. Do not let them dry out.

5. Serve with fresh chopped tomatoes and a drizzle of olive oil.

#16 Paleo Bacon Brussels Sprouts with a Twist

Yes, I admit it, I love bacon! The good thing about Paleo is that you don't have to give it up. Quite on the contrary: include more of it. The reason why bacon is criticized by many health watchers is that oftentimes it is accompanied by unhealthy processed foods like white bread, butter, and crisps. These must go, of course, because they are not within the Paleo lifestyle. However, adding bacon to some veggies is a different story. You can satisfy your bacon hunger and keep healthy and slim and the same time. Moreover, this dish is pretty alkaline as well. Not super alkaline, of course, but mildly. To be honest, I think that Brussels sprouts are boring, and that is why I add bacon and make it one of my preferred dishes. The total preparation time here is nearly an hour, so I suggest you keep it a dish for family and friends and get someone to help you.

Servings – 2

Ingredients

- ¼ cup of bacon, cut into strips or diced in small pieces

- 2 shallots or 1 small onion, chopped

- 2 cups Brussels sprouts, cleaned and cut in half

- ½ to 1 cup chestnuts, roasted and peeled

- Fresh thyme leaves

- ¼ cup chicken broth

- Salt and pepper, to taste

Instructions

1. Preheat oven to 220 degrees Celsius (430 Fahrenheit)

2. In the meantime, fry the bacon in a frying pan until it's crispy

3. Add the shallots and sauté for about 2 minutes until translucent. Add some broth if necessary.

4. Increase the heat and add the cabbage, sprouts, chestnuts, thyme, and broth, season and stir well with a wooden spoon.

5. Put skillet (or ovenproof pot that you used to stir-fry the ingredients) in the oven for about 25 minutes, stirring halfway through cooking with a spoon, until the sprouts are tender.

6. Serve immediately.

#17 Mini-Recipe: Guacamole and Bacon

Total Time - 10 minutes

Servings - 2 to 3

Ingredients

- 2 ripe avocados
- ½ medium red onion, chopped (or 2 scallions)
- A few sprigs of fresh cilantro, finely chopped
- Juice of half a lime
- 3 strips of bacon, cooked until they are crisp, crumbled
- 2 teaspoons spice mixture Merkén, or chili powder, or a pinch of ground coriander
- ½ ripe tomato, diced (Optional)
- Salt

Instructions

1. Mix all ingredients, except salt, mashing the avocado with a fork.

2. Try the guacamole and adjust salt to taste, add the spices.

3. Serve to accompany some sticks of raw vegetables or paleo gluten-free crackers.

#18.Creamy Bolognese Sauce

I love Italian food! The good news is that you can paleo-lize it and make it healthy. This recipe traditionally includes cheese, however, we will replace it with some almond powder (vegan cheese!). The spices remain the same, so your taste buds will be satisfied!

Total Prep Time: 2 hours 25 minutes

Servings - 6

Ingredients:

- 150g (about ½ cup) dried porcini

- 1 to 2 stalks celery

- 1 medium onion

- 3 carrots

- 1 red pepper

- 4-6 cloves of garlic

- 2 tablespoons coconut oil

- 2 sprigs rosemary

- 2 bay leaves

- 500g (2 cups) minced meat (I used 100% organic beef, but it could be mixed with chicken or pork)

- 250ml (1 cup) coconut milk

- 3 cups crushed tomatoes

- 1 cup beef stock

- Salt

- Pepper

- Crushed almonds (optional)

Instructions

1. Put the mushrooms in a bowl with boiling water and leave for about 15 minutes to rehydrate, then drain the mushrooms.

2. Chop the remaining vegetables and place in a food processor along with the mushrooms. Process to a smooth paste.

3. Heat some olive or coconut oil in a pan over medium heat, then add rosemary and bay leaf. Add the mushroom paste and fry for about 10 minutes. Keep stirring.

4. Increase the heat and add the meat.

5. Add the coconut milk and cook for 5-10 minutes until thickened. Coconut milk will make it creamy in a paleo way.

6. Add the crushed tomatoes, broth, salt, and pepper. Lower the heat and let it simmer for about 2 hours, stirring occasionally.

7. Serve with spaghetti of zucchini, squash, roasted sweet potatoes, or other vegetables. If you want an occasional cheat, you may sprinkle over some parmesan cheese. If you do paleo full-time, like me, then add some vegan almond cheese.

Enjoy!

#19.Classic Paleo Breakfast

There are many varieties of paleo omelettes. This is how I do it.

Servings - 2

Ingredients:

- 4 eggs (organic, free-range)

- 1 tablespoon organic olive oil

- 1 cup of spinach leaves (chopped finely)

-Fresh basil, chopped

- 1 small avocado

- Black pepper

Preparation:

1. Beat eggs in a small bowl.

2. Heat oil in a frying pan (medium heat is recommended) and add the eggs.

3. When the eggs are almost done, put the spinach on the top of one side. Add some basil and pepper, then fold in half.

4. Reduce heat and let it simmer for 1 minute.

5. Finally, garnish with some avocado slices.

Enjoy and have a powerful day!

#20. Jamaican Palaeolithic Twist

This is a really nice, spicy, tropical, paleo-friendly meal. Great for dinners with friends!

Servings - 4

Ingredients

- 4 tablespoons olive or coconut oil

- 2 cloves garlic, crushed

- 2 tablespoons fresh lemon juice

-1 teaspoon chili powder

- 1 teaspoon cumin

- 2 pounds flank steak, cut into strips

- 1 onion, cut into small pieces

- 1 red pepper, chopped

- 1 yellow pepper, cut into strips

- 1 tomato

- 2 tablespoons of dark rum (not really Paleo, but...!)

- ¼ cup fresh cilantro, chopped

Preparation

1. Place sliced steak in the bottom of a shallow glass dish.

2. Mix 2 tablespoons of olive oil with some garlic and lemon juice. Add some chili powder and cumin and shake the mixture to coat the steak.

3. Marinate the meat for about 2 hours (leave in the fridge).

4. Heat 1 tablespoon of your chosen cooking oil (coconut or olive) in a skillet over medium heat.

5. Add beef strips with any excess marinade and stir-fry.

6. Add the chopped onion and peppers and keep frying. Stir regularly.

7. Mix tomatoes (peeled and smashed) and rum. I suggest you use a blender or a food processor. Add to your veggies for extra taste and cook for about a minute.

8. Sprinkle with cilantro. Remove from heat and allow to cool.

#21.Cherry Berry Paleo Delight

Craving for sweets? Go for natural, Paleo-friendly choices.

Servings - 4

Ingredients:

- ½ cup Bing or Rainier cherries, pitted and chopped

- ½ cup blueberries

- 1 cup golden raspberries

- 1 cup blackberries

- 1 tsp. sweet almond powder

- ½ tsp. clove powder

- ½ cup cinnamon

- Handful of mint leaves

- Cocoa powder

Preparation:

1. Mix the cherries and berries in a bowl.

2. Add almond powder, clove, cinnamon, and fresh mint (chopped).
   3. Serve chilled.

3. Garnish with cocoa powder, nuts, or mint.

Yummy! My kids love it!

22. Confetti Rice Salad with Salmon

Servings: 2
Preparation time: 5-10 minutes

Ingredients:

- 1 cup of steamed cauliflower rice
- 3-4 oz. (113.4 grams) of cooked salmon
- 1/3rd cup of artichoke hearts
- 4 teaspoons of paleo mayonnaise
- 2 teaspoons of toasted cashew nuts
- 4 teaspoons of paleo white balsamic vinegar
- 1 cup celery, finely sliced
- 1 teaspoon of extra virgin olive oil
- 1/3rd cup of thinly sliced red or orange bell peppers
- 1/4th teaspoon of dry thyme
- 1.5 teaspoons of curry powder
- 11 whole scallion, sliced
- A pinch of Himalaya salt
- Fresh ground black pepper, according to taste

Method of preparation:

1. Whisk together thyme, paleo mayonnaise, balsamic vinegar, curry powder, olive oil and a pinch of salt. Set aside.
2. Add the scallions, artichoke hearts, bell pepper slices, celery slices, salmon and cashews with the cauliflower rice.
3. Add the mayonnaise dressing and toss again before serving to make sure it's equally spread on all the ingredients. Enjoy!

23. Apple Pecan Tuna Salad

Servings: 2-3
Preparation time: 10 minutes

Ingredients:

- 1 can of drained tuna
- 3 tablespoons of pecans
- 1/2 an apple, diced
- 1-2 tablespoons coconut yogurt
- 1/2 a stalk of celery, diced
- Ground black pepper, as required
- 1/2 lemon, juiced
- Sea salt, to taste

Method of preparation:

1. Chop the fruits and vegetables as is instructed and put in a bowl.
2. Add the remaining ingredients and stir well to combine. Serve and enjoy! I love coconut yoghurt or coconut milk (a nice alternative if you can't find coconut yoghurt) in my salads!

#24. Shrimp-Stuffed Avocados

Attention, seafood lovers! You can find something you like in the Paleo lifestyle since seafood plays a crucial role in it. Seafood is a great, healthy source of protein that is low-fat and rich in omega oils. All the things we need to make sure that our body and mind function at their optimal levels.

I love this recipe as a healthy snack.

Prep time - 5 minutes   *Servings - 4*

Ingredients:

- 4 large, peeled avocados (remove the seed and cut in half)

- 2 cups of shrimp (cooked, peeled, and ready to eat)

- 1 tbsp. fresh lemon juice

- 1 tbsp. onion powder

- 1 tsp. black pepper

- 1 tbsp. paprika

Preparation:

1. Put avocados in a bowl. The inside should be facing up (remove the seed of course).

2. Mix the shrimp with some lemon juice. Add onions and pepper (chopped).

3. Place shrimp mixture into each avocado, covering it as much as you can

4. Sprinkle the top of each stuffed avocado with paprika before serving.

Enjoy!

#25. Paleo-ized Chicken and Vegetable Soup

This is one of my favorite dishes for cold winters. It is also a great, natural remedy for colds and flu. I got this recipe from my wife, but of course, I had to add some chicken to make it suitable for carnivorous paleos!

Servings - 6

Ingredients:

- 6 cups water (filtered)

- A whole chicken, cut into cubes

- 2 cloves garlic, minced

- 1 yellow onion, chopped

- 1 bay leaf

- 1 tsp. black pepper

- 6 fresh tomatoes, diced

- 2 small zucchini, thinly sliced

- 3 carrots, diced

Preparation:

1. Mix some water with the chicken, garlic, and onion. Add bay leaf and pepper to spice it up.

2. Bring to a boil over medium heat.

3. Leave it on low about 2 hours, make sure that the chicken is tender.

4. Finally, add the remaining ingredients. Simmer for a few minutes.

5. Reduce heat.

6. 6. Cover and let it simmer for about 10 minutes or more. Check if the veggies are tender.

Serve warm, enjoy!

Algae is great natural source of many macronutrients that our modern, standard diet very often lacks. Even if you think you are healthy and eat lots of fruits and veggies, there is still something that you can improve.

I made sure that all my recipes taste great, so don't be put off by algae!

#26. Beet Soup and Alga Dulse

Ingredients:

- Dulse seaweed, powdered or cut (about 1-2 tbsp.)

- 2 cups red beets

- 1 cup coconut milk

- 1 clove garlic

- Juice of one fresh lemon

- White pepper

- Herbal salt

- Chopped chives

Preparation

1. Wash the beets and cook in boiling water so that the skin can be easily removed.

2. Drain and mix the beets with 1 cup of coconut milk.

3. Blend with the rest of the ingredients and dulse seaweed.

4. Add some lemon juice.

Optional: I love adding some nuts to this recipe.

#27. Avocado Salad with Sea Spaghetti Alga

Salads are easy and quick to prepare. Your imagination is the only limit of what can be created.

Servings - 4

Ingredients:

- 1 tbsp. Sea Spaghetti seaweed

- 4 avocados

- 2 carrots

- A handful of currants

- Olive oil

- Lemon

- Basil

Preparation:

1. Let the Sea Spaghetti soak in water for 20 minutes.
2. Peel avocados and cut them into thin slices. I suggest you spray them with lemon or lime so that they keep their natural color.
3. Wash and peel the carrots. Cut them into sticks.
4. Once the Sea Spaghetti is soaked, drain it and assemble the salad.
5. Here is how I normally organize the layout: a few drops of lemon first, followed by Sea Spaghetti, then avocados with carrots, then currants and some olive oil. To garnish, sprinkle it with some fresh basil.
6. Enjoy!

#28. Sugar and Fructose-free Apple Paleo Agar-Agar Dream Dessert

Ingredients:

- 2 tbsp. agar-agar

- ½ cup prunes (pitted)

- 6 apples

- Juice of half a lemon

- 3 tbsp. cream, almond puree, or crushed almonds

Preparation:

1. First, soak the sliced plums in filtered water. Next, add the agar-agar to soak and take on some nice flavor.

2. Meanwhile, peel and chop the apples and cook them for about 15 minutes over medium heat. Then, process them through a blender, adding agar-agar and plums. It's easier to achieve a nice, smooth, and thin cream when the apples are slightly cooked. I also suggest you keep the apple-infused water as it is full of minerals and vitamins.

3. Pour this mixture into a mold. Let it cool down.

4. Serve chilled, garnished with thin slices of green apple and a few drops of lemon juice.

5. Add some fresh mint and cinnamon if you like.

Enjoy!

#29. Seaweed Salad and Avocado

This is a super-quick and easy prep dish.

Servings - 3

Ingredients:

- 1 sheet of sea lettuce

- 2 avocadoes

- Juice of one lemon

- Olive oil

- 1 garlic clove

- 4 tomatoes

- 2 cucumbers

- 4 carrots

Preparation:

1. Soak the sea lettuce in filtered water for about 15 minutes.

2. In the meantime, peel and cut avocados, cucumbers, carrots, and garlic into small pieces.

3. Drain the soaked algae and mix with the veggies.

4. Sprinkle with some fresh lemon juice and olive oil.

5. Serve immediately.

#30. Kiwi-Wakame Paleo Smoothie

Wakame is my favorite algae. I like using it in my smoothies, too.

Preparation Time - 10 minutes

Servings - 2

Ingredients:

- 2 kiwis

- Juice of 2 lemons

- 2 bananas

- 1 small piece of ginger

- About 2 square inches of wakame (cut it out from wakame sheet)

- Coconut milk, half glass

- ½ glass water

- ½ teaspoon of chlorella powder (extra energy!)

Instructions:

1. Soak wakame in cold water for about 15 minutes.

2. In the meantime, peel and slice the kiwis and bananas, add them to a blender, and squeeze the lemon juice.

3. Blend all the ingredients and don't forget to add some chlorella powder.

Chlorella helped my wife and I quit coffee. If you are a coffee lover, try this recipe in the morning. Your energy will be restored naturally. Lemon juice stimulates the lymphatic system, which is a bit sluggish first thing in the morning, hence the feeling of heaviness, tiredness, and puffiness under the eyes.

#31. Japanese Paleo Twist

Another light Paleo option inspired by Japanese cuisine!

Preparation time - 25 minutes

Servings - 2

Ingredients:

- 1 tbsp. dried wakame seaweed

- 1 small cucumber

- 1 tbsp. olive oil

- A few drops of lemon juice

- 1-2 tsp. sesame seeds

- 1 pinch of sugar

- 1 small chili

Preparation:

1. Cover the dried wakame seaweed in warm filtered water. Leave to soak between 10 and 20 minutes. Then, drain and rinse in filtered water.

2. Peel the cucumber and cut into thin sticks. Lightly toast sesame seeds. Chop the chili and remove the seeds.

3. Mix the olive oil, sugar, and lemon juice in a bowl. Add the sesame and chili. Mix the seaweed with sliced cucumber.

4. Top seaweed and cucumber with the dressing.

This is a really light, refreshing Asian Paleo menu!

#32 Weight Loss Paleo Apple Pudding

Ingredients:

- Fresh, organic apples of your choice (about 1-2 kilos, it's up to you, I like cooking in bulk)
- 1 tbsp. vanilla powder
- Cinnamon (ground)
- One lemon (we will only need the zest, but you can also use add some of the juice to this pudding)
- Juice of 2 oranges
- 1 cup coconut milk
- 2 tbsp. powdered agar-agar

Preparation:

1. Wash and peel the apples. Cut them into small pieces and simmer them until soft.

2. Drain the apples, add the rest of the ingredients, and blend them.

3. Bake in the oven (180 degrees Celsius/350 Fahrenheit) until golden brown.

4. Allow to cool and put in the fridge

Serve cold with some cinnamon or fresh fruits. Enjoy!

Agar-agar is an algae full of nutrients and minerals. It also makes you feel full faster and prevents unhealthy food cravings. This is why I recommend it for weight loss regimes.

#33. Paleo Hijiki Time

Ingredients

- ½ cup hijiki seaweed, soaked about 20 minutes
- 1 large carrot, chopped into fine pieces
- ½ cup cooked sweet corn.
- 3 tbsp. walnuts, peeled and chopped
- A pinch of oregano.
- Olive oil.
- 1 cup alfalfa sprouts

Preparation:

1. 1. Boil the soaked and drained hijiki seaweed for about 20 minutes with 2 cups of water.

2. Add the carrots and olive oil, cook until the water is absorbed.

3. Allow to cool down.

4. Add sweet corn, nuts, oregano, and alfalfa sprouts.

#34. Paleo Seaweed Spaghetti

Servings - 1 to 2

Prep time - 30 minutes

Ingredients:

- 1 tbsp. Sea Spaghetti seaweed

- 1 zucchini, sliced

- 2 carrots, cut into thin strips

- 1 cabbage, finely sliced

- 1 small onion, finely chopped

- Olive oil

- Pepper

- Salt

Preparation:

1. Leave the Sea Spaghetti seaweed to soak for about 20 minutes (use warm filtered water).

2. Drain the Sea Spaghetti seaweed. Fry in some olive oil in a pan over low heat and add carrots and zucchini.

3. Keep stirring and frying.

4. After a couple of minutes, add the cabbage, onion, pepper, and salt.

I like to add a teaspoon of coconut oil near the end and love the way it tastes.

Serve immediately!

#35. Wakame Seaweed Salad

Servings - 2

Ingredients:

- 1 tbsp. wakame seaweed

- 1 cucumber

- 1 tsp. almond milk

- 1 tsp. coconut oil

- 1 tsp. sesame seeds

- 1 small chili (optional)

Preparation:

1. Let the seaweed soak in warm filtered water for about 15 minutes. Then drain, rinse, and set aside.

2. Peel the cucumber and slice into thin pieces. Toast the sesame seeds and mince some chilli if you like your food spicy.

3. Add the algae and put everything together in a salad bowl.

4. Dressing: In a small bowl, mix the coconut oil, sweet almond oil, and lemon juice. Add the sesame and diced chili pepper and mix.

Serve immediately. Enjoy!

#36. Paleo Sardines Like Whiskey!

Prep time: 7 minutes

Servings - 2

Ingredients:

- 4 sardines

- 1 tbsp. dried alga dulse

- 1 tbsp. whiskey

- ½ glass of coconut milk

- 10 cherry tomatoes (peeled and seeded)

- 2 tbsp. coconut oil

- 1 lemon

Preparation:

1. Soak the alga dulse in filtered water for about 15 minutes. Then drain, rinse, and set aside.

2. Put soaked alga dulse in a blender and add the other ingredients. Blend. Taste and add some salt if necessary.

3. Serve the sardines with the sauce and half of a lemon to garnish. Sprinkle the dish with fresh lemon juice if necessary.

Enjoy! This is a delicious snack!

#37. Easy Seaweed Salad

Servings - 2

Ingredients:

- 1 handful wakame

-1 handful hijiki seaweed

-1 handful Atlantic dulse

- 4 baby carrots

- 2 tbsp. peanuts

- 2 tbsp. olive oil

- 2 tbsp. orange juice

- Salt and pepper

Preparation:

1. Pour all the seaweed in a pot filled with warm water and leave to soak for 10 minutes.

2. In the meantime, wash, peel, and chop the carrots.

3. Mix all the ingredients in a bowl and add some olive oil, orange juice, salt, and pepper.

#38. Fishy Paleolithic Taste

Servings - 4

Ingredients:

- 3 cups fish stock

-1 cup sweet potatoes

- 2 tbsp. mild olive oil

- 1 cucumber

- 3 tbsp. various algae or seaweed (Irish moss, sea lettuce, sea spaghetti, etc.)

- ½ red and green pepper

- ½ red onion

- Handful of chopped chives

- 30ml extra virgin olive oil

Preparation:

1. Wash and peel the potatoes and boil them in the fish stock.

2. Once cooked, process them in a blender. Add some mild olive oil to help achieve the desired texture. Set aside, then chill in the fridge

3. Wash and chop other ingredients and put them in a separate bowl. Add the seaweed and sprinkle with extra virgin oil.

4. Add the cold, creamy potato sauce.

5. Garnish with chopped chives.

Serve nicely chilled! Enjoy!

#39. Paleo Tuna with Algae

Servings - 4

Ingredients:

- 4 tuna steaks

- Sesame oil

- 1 hazelnut-sized piece of ginger root

- Extra virgin olive oil

- 2 tbsp. dried sea spaghetti

- 1 red pepper

- 2 zucchini

- 2 cloves of garlic

- Salt

- ½ cup coconut milk

Preparation:

1. Marinate the tuna with some ginger, a pinch of salt, olive oil, and garlic. Leave in the fridge for about half an hour. Do not leave it in for too long.

2. In the meantime, prepare the algae. Soak it in warm filtered water for about 20 minutes.

3. Prepare the veggies. Cut into small pieces and stir-fry on low heat together with some garlic. Then add the soaked algae and stir-fry until a saucy consistency is achieved. Blend and add some coconut milk for creamy consistency.

4. Serve the tuna warm or chilled with this delicious, creamy sauce that is rich in minerals.

5. Garnish with ginger paste (I usually blend ginger with some coconut milk).

Don't forget to pick up your free complimentary PDF eBook available at:

www.HolisticWellnessBooks.com/bonus

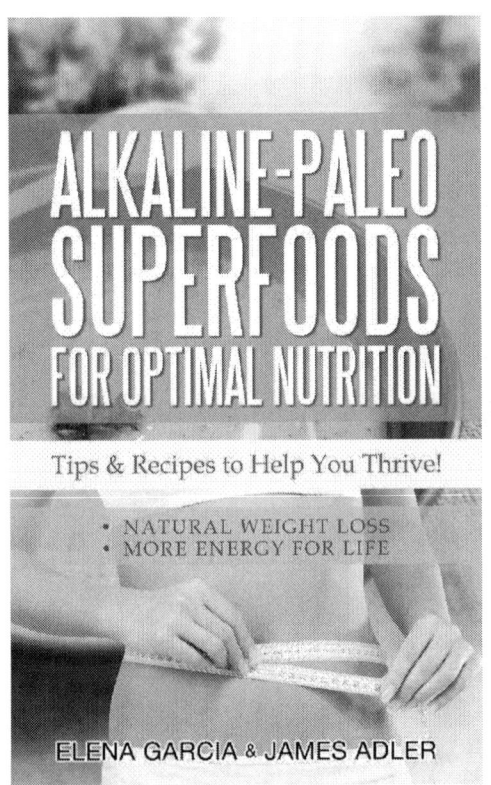

#40. Sexy Skinny

Servings - 2 to 3

Ingredients:

- 1 small broccoli

- 1 small cauliflower

- 2 eggs

- Olive oil

- 1 lemon

- Paprika

Preparation:

1. Boil the broccoli and cauliflower for a few minutes over medium heat to soften them. You don't want them to cook too much.

2. In the meantime, prepare the paleo mayo. Blend one egg with some olive oil and a squeeze of fresh lemon juice. Then add some paprika. Whisk until it starts to become thick.

3. Drain the veggies. Keep the water for soups and other recipes, it's full of minerals and vitamins! Put the veggies in the bottom of a baking dish. Cover with our paleo mayonnaise.

4. Bake in the oven (180 Celsius or 350 Fahrenheit) until slightly brownish.

I like to garnish it with some chopped onions, radish, and parsley.

This is how my kids fell in love with broccoli!

Serve immediately. Enjoy!

Chapter 7 Paleo Motivation for a Lifetime

Paleo is not just a diet, **it is a lifestyle**. Yet, because it is a different lifestyle than most of our society chooses to adopt, it takes **motivation** to continue at it for a lifetime.

Most of my motivation comes from the results I have seen in my own life thanks to Paleo. I have more energy than ever. I have been able to maintain a lean and healthy body. The ailments that plagued me for so long have vanished. This is basically my main motivation. Why wouldn't I want to continue to have all of these things by living a Paleo life?

Write down what you wanted to achieve when you're starting Paleo. What is the goal?

– To be healthy?

– To be lean?

– To be free of disease and allergies?

Update what you want to achieve on a semi-regular basis. Evaluate on a regular basis whether or not you have gained or achieved your goal, and keep the focus on how happy you are with your new life. Always read it when you feel your resolve fading.

Keep your Paleo diet interesting. That is something that helped me immensely. Use different methods to cook your meats and vegetables: grilling, braising, sautéing, stir-frying, roasting, slow cooking, steaming, broiling, and poaching are all awesome ways to keep variety in your meals in order to stay motivated.

Mimic techniques that restaurants use to create an eating experience as opposed to just a meal. It helps me to enjoy my food rather than just having something to eat. Here are some ways to create your own eating experience:

-Use garnish! You can make a beautiful presentation on your plate in your own kitchen.

- Turn a boring serving of food into a beautiful meal that you can enjoy. Instead of throwing salad into a bowl, put it on your plate.

- Use a variety of colors when choosing salad ingredients and arrange them on a plate with a decorative drizzle of dressing.

- Instead of piling vegetables next to a piece of meat, make an arrangement around the meat or pour them over the top. An edible art piece!

- Garnishes can be part of the meal. Use roasted nuts, citrus fruits sliced into swirls, or fresh herbs.

- Use a beautiful table setting to make your meal more inviting. Choose a good combination of prints and colors.

- Visit a thrift store and find some vintage plates, serving bowls, or glasses to make an everyday dinner feel special.

- Put a pitcher of water on your table to bring the restaurant-feel to your home.

- Add lemon, lime, mint, or cucumber to your water glasses. It makes your beverage healthier and more inviting.

- Eating in courses is not just for eating out or a holiday meal. Try it every day. Take time to enjoy an appetizer or salad before bringing out the main dish. Take a few minutes between courses like you would when dining out. The longer you take to enjoy your food, the easier it is for your brain to recognize that it is full. You will eat less while enjoying yourself more.

These tips are only a few of the ways you can keep yourself motivated as you continue in your healthy Paleo lifestyle. My main motivation is found in my results. The most beautiful part of result-based motivation is that it is right there with me all the time.

The Paleo diet can be also successfully combined with the alkaline diet.

We have a free PDF guide that you can get at:

www.holisticwellnessbooks.com/bonus

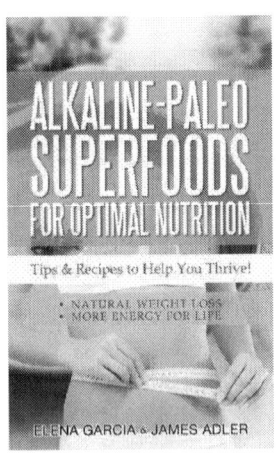

If you happen to have any problems with your download, email us at:

info@holisticwellnessbooks.com

Bonus Chapter: NLP for Weight Loss

NLP Techniques for Successful Weight Loss?

I hope that this chapter will provide you with some additional weight loss motivation tools that come from Neuro-Linguistic Programming (NLP). There is no theory here, only some practical examples for you to start applying.

Thanks to a **boosted motivation level**, I was on my way to the "new me." At the beginning of the process, I realized that every day, I felt as if I was battling my old eating habits. I would over-eat. Consuming more calories than I was burning was stifling my goal. Eating the wrong foods was also keeping me from achieving physical wellbeing. I used a specific technique to change my bad eating habits, a technique referred to as the Swish Pattern.

The **Swish Pattern** is a useful tool in changing old bad habits easily. It is a technique where you replace an undesirable habit with one you would prefer to have. I wanted to replace my unhealthy eating habits (like junk food and over-eating) with healthy eating habits (like choosing energizing foods and eating healthy portions). This tool helped me change my thoughts and thought process regarding these habits, which in turn changed the bad behavior.

SWISH PATTERN

First, choose the habit or behavior that you want to replace. Visualize it in your mind. Be in the moment of acting out this behavior. Use your five senses to recognize exactly what it feels like. What emotions do you have? Isolate a certain, vividly detailed image of yourself in the midst of engaging in this habit. For me, it was imagining myself shoving pizza into my mouth. Make sure you recognize that this is something you have done in the past and that you want to keep it there. Take a mental picture.

Next, using all of your senses again, create another image of yourself being successful by replacing that bad eating habit with a healthy one. This will be your replacement snap shot. It is vivid, intense, and vibrant. In mine, I had eaten well and used proper portions. I was healthy and energized thanks to making good choices in regard to food. Step outside of the picture to see yourself in it. At the bottom corner of the new image, you will place a tiny version of yourself in the midst of your bad habit. This tiny picture is dark and colorless.

A healthy and balanced meal, or...

Indulging in unhealthy habits?

Now, re-visualize the first picture, the old you. At the bottom corner, darken the future picture (of you and your replacement behavior) and make it small. You can still see it, but it is darker. Put yourself back into the poor emotional state that you are currently in. This is currently the big image. You should be feeling all of the self-defeating emotions associated with your bad habit like disappointment and self-loathing. Fully connect yourself with that moment.

Now, instantaneously switch the two images. Bring back the "new you," with your replacement behavior. Make it huge and colorful, full of everything to stimulate your senses. Shrink the picture of your unwanted behavior at the same time, moving it back into the corner and darkening it. When you do this, make a "swishhh" sound. As I did this, I would mentally jump into the replacement behavior image. The picture of you in the future is now the present. The old behavior is in the past, exactly where you want it to be.

I repeated this several times. Switching the pictures and jumping into my new behavioral image while "swishing." Gradually increase the speed of the switch. Eventually, it will become instantaneous. Replacing your bad eating habit will be as simple as that.

SETTING AN ANCHOR

Another Neuro-linguistic Programming technique I used on a consistent basis during my weight loss journey was Anchoring. Setting an anchor was immensely beneficial to me, and I hope that it is for you as well. It helped me to get back the feeling of being motivated, healthy, and happy like I used to be when I was in shape and healthy years ago. This technique helped to keep me driven during my weight loss program. The beauty of this process is that if one anchor does not produce the results you are looking for, it can always be replaced.

Anchoring Facts:

- They can be produced artificially or naturally (due to events).

- They can occur because of a single emotionally-charged event or subconsciously through repetition, for example advertising.

- Needs to be repeated; it can fade with time.

- Make sure you set the anchor when the feeling you want to reinforce is at its peak.

- Choose a very intense memory.

- Make sure that the stimulus you are using is as exclusive as possible. Don't use something you do all the time.

- I stacked (set) my anchors for approximately 30 minutes; the longer the duration of repetition, the better.

1. **Choosing a memory** - I remembered a time I was at the gym and was asked to be a trainer because I was at my physical best. You choose your own. Make sure it was emotionally intense.

2. **Reliving the memory** - Associate yourself with the memory. Be in that moment and see it through your own eyes. This made my feelings more intense. I made the picture of the event extremely colorful, large, and bright. I intensified my feelings to the maximum.

3. **Anchoring the memory** - When I felt my emotions at their peak, I pinched the back of my hand. That was my trigger. You can do whatever works best for you: rub your earlobe, grab your knee, etc.

4. **Stop at your peak** - Release your trigger when your emotion peaks. I had to practice this step a few times before I had it down.

5. **Testing the trigger/anchor** - I stopped for a while and thought about something else, then used my trigger. If anchoring was successful, it will bring you back to that lovely emotional state immediately.

6. **Repeat** - Repeat this several times. To make my anchor stronger and more powerful, I set 3-4 memories of times when I felt the same way to that identical trigger.

Anchoring was the most effective ways to put myself in a motivated, positive mindset during my weight loss program. I used it almost every day, throughout the day. My trigger helped me be able to feel awesome and driven on demand. What better way to make it through a weight loss program?

SELF-CHECK

An additional way I used NLP ideas in my weight loss program was to check in with myself every day. I needed to make sure that I was staying on track. I would think about and ask myself these key questions:

1. What do I desire?

2. How will getting that help me?

3. What obstacles are keeping me from getting it?

4. What is essential to me?

5. What is working best in this situation?

6. What could be enhanced?

7. What resources am I going to utilize?

Self-evaluation is necessary to achieve any goal. Success in the short or long-term requires that questions be asked and answers be evaluated. Then, if necessary, redirection must occur.

Conclusion

Thank you again for taking an interest in this guide.

I hope it was able to help give you a solid beginning in understanding what the Paleo lifestyle is all about. It is not just a diet, it is a perspective on life and how to live it to the fullest. Paleo is not just the newest fad diet, it is the oldest, healthiest way to eat!

It is my desire that the recipes and tips included sparked something inside of you. **This is only the tip of the iceberg!** The more you learn, the more you will want to put it into practice.

I encourage you to jump right in and get started. You have nothing to lose but weight and health problems, and everything to gain: health, wellness, and vitality for the rest of your life!

We were biologically designed to process certain foods in order to maintain maximum health. I hope you have realized, as I did, that it is not a matter of failing at previous diets. "Diets" themselves are failures by design. The only way to achieve success is to model what has always been successful. For us as human beings, it is to eat as our ancient Paleolithic ancestors: free of disease, depression, allergies, and obesity.

I did it. I am doing it. You can too!

Finally, if you enjoyed this book, please take the time to share your thoughts and post a review. It would be greatly appreciated!

Thank you, and good luck!

James Adler

For similar books, please visit:

www.HolisticWellnessBooks.com

Also, before you go, remember to join our free newsletter and claim your free bonus PDF eBook as a welcome gift. It's waiting for you at:

www.HolisticWellnessBooks.com/bonus

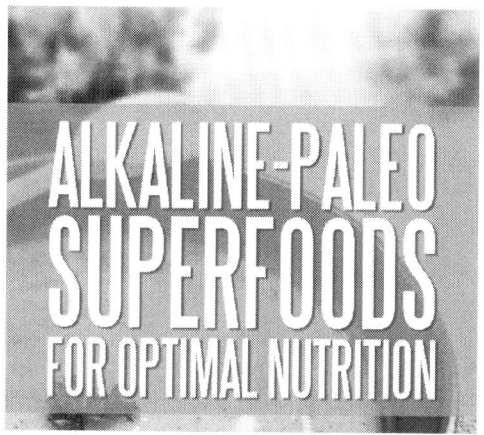
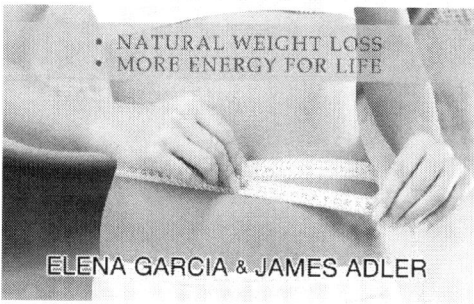

Any problems, please email us at:

info@holisticwellnessbooks.com

Printed in Great Britain
by Amazon

34868894R00052